The Calm Bladder

Freedom from cystitis

Dr Tim Whittlestone MA, MD
FRCS(Urol)

Consultant Urologist

ISBN: **978-1499622041**
ISBN-13: **149962204X**

IS THIS BOOK FOR YOU?

Are you plagued with recurrent bladder infections? Does your bladder rule your life? Have you been diagnosed with cystitis, interstitial cystitis or recurrent UTI? Then this is the book for you.

The content is primarily designed for sufferers of cystitis and recurrent cystitis symptoms. We will touch upon interstitial cystitis and non – infective causes of bladder symptoms. There is advice for both men and women.

I have written this book with the patient in mind although I haven't been frightened to use medical terms. Many of my patients with bladder symptoms have seen healthcare professionals before and most understand the terms. I also hope that this is useful for doctors, nurses and carers of those with bladder symptoms. There is much ignorance in this subject field and much for all of us to learn and share.

The advice in this book is not intended to substitute medical care. You should always see a doctor before embarking on treatment.

Tim Whittlestone

CONTENTS

ACKNOWLEDGMENTS

This book could only have been put together with the help and support of the thousands of patients I've met with bladder symptoms. Seeing your lives transformed has encouraged me to offer some of our tips to a wider audience. Thank you!

1 THE BLADDER

The Bladder is a floppy bag of muscle that sits deep within the pelvis and holds about 400mls of fluid. Its job is simple. To Store and expel urine. At birth, just like non-humans, the bladder fills up with wee minute by minute. When it reaches its capacity a signal from the bladder fires in the spinal cord and it switches from its STORE function to it's EXPEL role. Hence the baby urinates anytime, day or night. Given that humans are generally embarrassed by watching each other pee, we have learnt to ignore the signals from the full bladder and instead find a socially appropriate location to expel our waste. This is bladder training, a lesson that we teach very poorly, and a subject that I will return to again and again.

Now the bladder is not perfectly formed. For starters it has to share the pelvis with lots of odd structures – the bowel, the womb, the ovaries just to name a few. A consequence of this is that illness on one of these neighborhood structures will have knock on effects on the bladder and vice versa. It's a common scenario that the inflammation in the colon which accompanies gastroenteritis, for example, will spill over to the bladder and give symptoms of cystitis. And it follows that a bladder infection will upset your bowels!

The next design flaw has its roots in the complex science of embryology. If you start with the mental image of a flat plate of cells, then start to roll up that sheet and crumple up the ends you'll form a cylinder. This is the basis of the human fetus and every organ contained within. So the bladder starts flat and ends up a hollow ball. Great, but.... Some parts of the ball are from a different set of crockery! The bladder base is made from, a whole different set of cells, with different properties and skills than the rest of the organ. These cells seem to be more like skin cells, rough and flaky, whereas the remainder of the bladder has a silky smooth, non-stick surface. Whatever your personal theory on the genesis of humankind, design features like this one leave us with problems. Rough and flaky is perfect breeding ground for bacteria!

Most of us have seen the naked opposite sex and the differences between man and woman. The penis is a great extension of the bladder and provides it with an extra 15 or so centimeters of distance from the outside world. The poor female bladder is woefully exposed being 2-3 centimeters from the filthy environment in which we live. Bugs have an innate ability to stroll, climb and permeate the body's natural orifices. The female bladder is constantly invaded by bacteria, yeasts and viruses. It's no fault of hygiene, just a plane old fact of life, that the bladder becomes a melting pot of organisms.

It's helpful to start to examine the myriad of defence

mechanisms the human body has designed to prevent urinary infections. The mainstay of defence is the very action of peeing. I like to think about the kid's paddling pool out in the garden. Left undisturbed for a day or two its pretty ok. Then from day 3 it starts to looks less appealing. Dead flies, grass cuttings and an oily sun cream fill start to build up on the surface. A day or two more and the bird droppings look positively unwelcoming. The kids stop using it and the algae blooms around the edges, the flies begin the breed and eventually you have a health hazard. In the summer months we've learnt to empty it out daily and refill it when the sun comes out again. Same with the bladder!

The bladder can store wee for hours but eventually the urge to urinate becomes compelling. Micturition, the act of passing wee, is incredibly efficient allowing us to expel every last drop of urine from the bladder. And good job too as even small amounts of 'residual' urine, left behind after we think we've finished, can easily become the source of infection. So passing urine, just like emptying the paddling pool, is vital for health. Life, civilization, work, family and social attitudes have resulted in a negative impression of the common pee. We do it locked away, out of sight and treat it as a terrible inconvenience. In many respects bladder training has gone too far. Most of us would like to urinate as little as often so that we don't miss a vital part of the meeting or such that we don't need to turn off the road to find a toilet stop. By reducing the frequency of passing urine we are actually denying the bladder the simplest and most elegant form of natural defence. And it gets even worse! The pharmaceutical industry have hit on a gold mine in the manufacture and marketing of drugs that actually reduce the number of times we need to pee. Parents have been told to rigorously enforce bladder training for children as young as 2 in order to get them ready for out-of-home child care routines. And the very phrase 'weak bladder' implies someone who pees too often - a source of ridicule and humour.

Next defence in line is the bladder wall. I've explained that in its making in the fetus the bladder mainly derives form a shiny, flat walled plate of cells. This is good! The resulting bladder lining is effectively a non-stick pan, featureless and smooth. Pathogens (the bad guys) need to be able to settle in the bladder if they are going to breed, secrete toxic chemicals and generally make a nuisance of themselves. To do this they latch onto the surfaces of cells, often by means of fairly elaborate arms or tentacles. The flatter and smoother the cellular lining of an organ, the less able these tentacles are to grab hold and establish a colony. The gut lining is completely the opposite – all rough and pot holed. In that way the gut actually encourages bacteria and yeasts to live and grow in its lumen, harnessing the bugs for beneficial effects.

The bladder goes even further with this defence strategy. The smooth cells produce chemicals and proteins that stick to the bacterial tentacles and confuse them! Once these chemicals bind with the bug's arms then they are useless at sticking to the bladder lining. It's rather like flack fired into the sky to confuse the enemy aircraft and its incredibly effective. Or at least it would be if we all produced it! Unfortunately about 1 in 10 of us have a genetic variation that stops us secreting these protective proteins.

Finally the urine itself offers us some protection from the invading bugs. The chemical composition varies hour to hour. The main constituent of urine is water but chemicals such as nitrogen and ammonia make it difficult for pathogens to survive. Urine has been studied for millennia. The Greeks wrote books on it, the Romans were mesmerized by it and early medicine analyzed it to exhaustion. Doctors and amateur physicians have been extolling the virtues of the acid urine or the alkaline urine for over 200 years. The truth is that urine pH varies wildly and is most commonly neutral (neither acid nor alkaline). It's the neutrality of the urine that offers protection from bacterial growth. We've been wasting our time trying to change the pH of urine, lost in some belief that making it 'more acid' would kill of bugs. The cranberry farmers have done well!

2 THE SCOPE OF THE PROBLEM

It's reassuring that your are never alone when it comes to cystitis. In actually fact you've chosen the second commonest complaint of patients in the waiting room of the average family doctor. You've exposed yourself to a multi million-dollar industry and joined the ranks of the 150 million patients reporting a urinary tract infection every year.

We estimate a lifetime risk of getting cystitis is close to 100% for women and 20% for men. Hang on! That means that every woman on the planet will get a urinary tract infection in her lifetime. Half of all women will suffer with recurrent infection – year after year. So common is the phenomenon of recurrent infection that the medical profession 'normalizes' cystitis – most doctors don't get excited if the frequency of infection is less that 3 episodes a year. And the stats tell us that 1 in 10 women get persistent infection with symptoms month-on-month.

Looked at another way, urinary tract infection accounts

for 400 million lost days work every year. It results in endless pain and suffering and is estimated to be a contributory factor in 90,000 deaths every year in the UK. The trouble with these statistics is that they woefully underestimate the truth. Either because many patients have lost faith in their medical system, or because they culturally and socially believe that cystitis is best kept quiet, the reporting of symptoms is way below the true picture.

We make it hard on ourselves to accept that the symptoms of urinary infection need attention. There is a popular misconception that cystitis is a disease of the unclean! Many people believe that cystitis is a sexually transmitted infection (it is not), or that if occurs as a result of poor personal hygiene (it does not). There is a stigma attached to bladder disease. Who has not heard of 'honeymoon cystitis'? I have heard women tell me that they probably caught cystitis because they slept with the wrong man, or that they accidently wore the same knickers two days in a row, or the classic case of the dirty toilet seat! It is outrageous that as a society we have allowed these beliefs to survive. We feel confident phoning our boss to excuse our absence for a chest infection but admitting to cystitis is tantamount to saying you've got syphilis! This behavior leads to underreporting. We have no idea about the true incidence of urinary infections in the general population. We know therefore that you are not alone; we predict that you have experienced one of the commonest ailments known to mankind – symptoms that practically everyone can sympathize with.

Where things get less common and more serious is the recurrent or persisting variety of urinary infection that starts as a bladder symptom and soon leads to a life less worth living.

It's useful at this point to see what we mean by the terms 'recurrent infection' and 'persisting infection'. A recurrent infection implies that the cystitis clears completely and then returns. In other words the individual concerned has symptoms of cystitis, the infection is treated by self help or medical intervention, the patient is then free of symptoms for a period and eventually the infection returns. The cycle goes on – infection – treatment – disease free – infection – treatment – disease free, etc. Common dogma dictates that more than 2 or 3 infections each twelve months implies recurrent infection. This is a dogma we will challenge later!

Persistent infection suggests that the cystitis never clears, that symptoms, whilst varying in intensity, are ever present. This is a confusing. We know that acute infection of the bladder with bacteria growing and proliferating can be treated in some people very rapidly with antibiotics. In some cases the drugs take only hours to work. The bacteria are killed or prevented from breeding and the bladder clears the bugs from the body. The symptoms of cystitis can, however, persist for days and weeks. The effect of infection is inflammation. You know inflammation as it's a common response of the body to disease. You've experienced inflammation around a sore spot or boil. You have felt the effects of inflammation on your skin after you've been burned by the sun. You can see inflammation in your eyes and around your nose when you've been exposed to pollen or cat hair. It is unpleasant. It's red. It's sore. And it lasts for days and weeks. This is exactly the same process which your bladder endures with cystitis. Urologists like me try to avoid looking inside the bladders of patients with infection for fear it will make the cystitis worse but when we do take a peek inside it can be shocking. The bladder wall is bright red, often with bleeding ulcers. The cellular lining of the bladder is swollen and puffy with fluid. And the patient, should they be awake during the procedure is in pain. Severe pain. It's like poking a patch of sunburn with a stick. Persistent infection is often confused with the after effects of acute cystitis – inflammation.

My own diagnosis of recurrent cystitis is based purely on observations of patients. If the sufferer tells me that BETWEEN episodes they are SYMPTOM FREE, can return to a normal existence and forget all about their bladder then I'm satisfied they have recurrent cystitis – no matter how many episodes they get over the year.

With persistent infection the diagnosis is based on urine tests. Clever chemists have invented tiny strips of plastic loaded with ten or so mini experiments. If the strip is dipped in urine then the chemistry magic occurs and indicates, by means of a colour change, the presence or absence of 10 substances in the bladder. These 'dipsticks' are universal, cheap and accurate. We can examine fresh urine with confidence and look for markers of inflammation and infection. In essence the bacteria that are mainly responsible for cystitis create NITRATES in the urine. If the symptoms of cystitis persist and the nitrates are ever present in the dipstick result then it's most likely a persisting infection. The urine dip test can reveal other abnormalities such as LEUCOCYTES (white blood cells) and RED BLOOD CELLS. These are markers of inflammation, not specifically for persisting infection. The presence of one or both of these markers on dip testing in an individual with persisting cystitis like symptoms (in the absence of the nitrates) suggests to me that it's inflammation, not infection that needs attention. The difference might seem subtle, but it does have huge implications for the treatment of the symptoms.

NITRATES +/- LEUCOCYTES +/- RED CELLS
= Infection + Inflammation

LEUCOYTES +/- RED CELLS
= Inflammation Alone

In my work as a urologist I see very little acute infection – the majority is dealt with by family doctors or treated at home by individuals using self help techniques. Of the thousands of patients I've seen referred to me, 60% have recurrent cystitis, 20% have persisting inflammation, 10% have persisting infection and the remainder have non-infective causes of their symptoms.

It's the last group, the non-infection patients, that offer the greatest challenge in diagnosis and treatment. Every year urologists will see men and women who have been treated for years for recurrent or persistent cystitis with multiple course of antibiotics but who have never experienced any significant improvement. In these we will diagnose various diseases including bladder cancer, bowel cancer, diverticular disease of the colon and interstitial cystitis.

Cancer diagnoses are, thankfully, rare. In general the persistent finding of blood in the urine – either visible blood or the red cells detected on the dipsticks – would alert me to the need for a cystoscopy (examination of the bladder lining with a camera). Other risk factors such as smoking, family history and exposure to certain dangerous chemicals (those used in the dye and paint industry including hair dyes) would increase my suspicion of cystitis bladder symptoms. Bowel cancer can result in persisting infection if the cancer grows into the bladder – remember that the poor bladder has to share a crowded pelvis. Eventually the cancer can erode into the bladder allowing the bacteria rich contents of the bowel easy passage into the bladder. The same can be true of diverticular disease – a condition currently enjoying a high prevalence in Western countries. With bowel disorders especially bowel cancers a change in bowel habit usually occurs – passing poo gets more or less frequent and it can be associated with mucus and blood on the toilet paper or in the toilet pan.

I couldn't write a book on the bladder without mentioning the condition of interstitial cystitis (IC). It's the rarest form of cystitis but it's the one which is practically impossible to cure. As such IC enjoys a fearful reputation, is over diagnosed and attracts a lot of media and internet attention. We don't know the cause so I can only speculate. If you recall the bladder lining is smooth and shiny. In order to achieve this the cells are packed together like crazy paving, the cells neatly and snugly arranged. There are no gaps, it's one continuous sheet. And that has advantages as the urine does some pretty noxious stuff. The gapless barrier of the bladder lining prevents urine from coming into contact with the delicate and complex deeper layers of the bladder which contain blood vessels, nerves and muscle cells. With IC we know that this barrier is breached, gaps do start to appear between cells and urine seeps into the deep layers. We have no idea what causes these gaps, maybe it's a genetic defect or perhaps an autoimmune phenomenon (where the body attacks it's own cells). Whatever the cause the result is patchy inflammation (again) of the bladder, pain and urinary symptoms that seem impossible to solve. There are some useful ways to diagnose IC – the appearance of the bladder at cystoscopy, the presence of ulcers within the bladder, the way the bladder reacts to being stretched and the presence of special cells (mast cells) within the bladder wall – that allow urologists to make the diagnosis usually with the aid of a bladder biopsy (removal of a tiny bit of bladder for analysis). I'll came back to IC in a chapter of it's own.

Men are a special case! It's much less common for a man to suffer cystitis – the penis offers natural protection. Sporadic infection occurs but there is often an underlying problem, mostly with the plumbing. We know that flushing out the bladder at regular intervals is a vital instrument of defence. When any, however small, volume of urine is retained in the bladder recurrent and persistent infections usually follow. Men have a prostate which grows with age. The effect of prostate growth is to narrow the exit of the bladder and impede its full and efficient emptying. The same is true for isolated narrowing of the water pipe as can occur following relatively minor trauma to the penis or insertion of instruments and catheters into the male bladder. Even slight narrowing of the urethra (water pipe) resulting in a subtle change to the force of peeing can result in recurrent cystitis. These effects mean that the men tend to be older than women when they present with cystitis. Furthermore, faulty plumbing is usually amenable to a simple fix. Urologist spend most of their days widening tubes or coring away prostate over growth.

Hopefully the scope of the problem is clear. It's a massive problem. All women get bladder infections and millions get recurrent and persisting symptoms caused either by infection of inflammation. IC is rare but awful. Men fair much better but can nevertheless be debilitated by the symptoms of cystitis. Lets move on to look at that range of symptoms in the next chapter.

3 SYMPTOMS

How do you know when you've got cystitis? Practically everyone can answer the question with 2 words – PAIN and FREQUENCY. These are indeed the 'classical' symptoms of infection. The pain comes from the inflammation – think sunburn again. The frequency means an increase in the number of times you feel you need to pee.

Remember how the bladder works – it stores urine most of the time and when its getting full it tells you its time to go. The nerves that sense pain and the ones that sense fullness are all co-located. Pain itself sends an impulse to the brain that we perceive as a full bladder. Our bladder training routine kicks in and we find a toilet. The same works in reverse – we all know that a very full bladder is painful. Despite the beauty of nature and the intricacies of the human body sometimes we just get these signals mixed up. And it does make sense that if we have something noxious in our bladder then we'd better try to expel it and vice versa what better way to grab your attention when your bladder is seriously full than a bit of pain!

Frequency is almost impossible to define. One of the commonest questions I'm asked as a urologist is 'how often should I need to urinate'? The answer varies widely, once a day, twenty times a day? It all comes back to bladder training. Schooling and the workplace have dictated that its reasonable to pee about 4 or 5 times a day – before you set off, at lunch beak, at the end of the school or work day and before bed. That's roughly every 4 hours. If urine is produced by the kidneys at a rate of 40 to 80 millilitres per hour then that equates to urine volumes of between 160 to 320 millilitres per pee. And actually that is just about what we find in detailed measurements across large numbers of humans. The bladder can hold more, much more urine if you try. It's a very flexible device. As the bladder stretches so it also relaxes. Over time individuals can train their bladder to hold litres of urine. There's no point in doing that and as you can imagine the consequences can be severe.

Equally bladder training can go the other way. Despite believing that its harmful in the long term I still instruct my children to go pee before a long car journey or before we board a plane. It's ingrained that somehow its impossible to stop mid journey, that the toilets will be dirty and smelly or that we can't be getting up too often in an aircraft. Equally one of the greatest fears of every human is that of wetting themselves in public. It's always there in the top ten lists of feared experience. How often have you seen someone wet themselves? Not that often I guess. We overplay the fear of involuntary loss of urine perhaps because humans have associated incontinence with some form of madness or insanity.

So bladder training results in a whole spectrum of 'normal' frequency and what is normal now may change for you in the future. If you change your lifestyle, change how much you drink or move on to a new job so your bladder frequency will change.

With cystitis there is almost a constant desire to pass urine. The inflammation doesn't go away with each pee and hence the confused signals keep escaping to your brain. It's not uncommon to want to pass urine every 20 minutes or so.

Another symptom, closely associated with frequency, is urgency. You want to go and you want to go now! The signals from the bladder telling you you've reached your personal capacity come along in trains, one after the other. The faster those signals arrive in the brain then the more urgently you need to pee. With infection and inflammation the signals are firing off repeatedly and urgency is a natural phenomenon. The worrying aspect of urgency is that at some point the signals are so rapid that you loose your willful control of the bladder. The bladder resorts to the that of the newborn baby and switches itself to expel mode – you do wet yourself.

So these are, in my mind, the classical symptoms of cystitis – pain, increase in urinary frequency and urgency to pass urine. But there are more, many more.

Let us examine pain. The pain of bladder inflammation can be manifest in numerous ways. Some patients find it painful to pass urine – this is because the highest concentration of the pain nerves are found around the base of the bladder and the beginning of the water pipe. As the urine flows over this region it contracts and worsens the pain. Pain can be referred – that is the origin of the pain can be confusing. With the bladder, pain can be experienced low down in the tummy – the suprapubic region, in the low spine area, in the tops of the legs/thighs and at the tip of the urethra. In men the pain of cystitis is often felt at the very tip of the penis, in women the tip of the urethra becomes sore making the vulva and vagina area seem at fault.

Pain can be specific – sometimes its possible to pin point the source (or apparent source) of the pain. Other times pain is vague, generalized and difficult to define to origin. 'Pelvic pain' is a broad term used to describe menstrual pain, the pain associated with ovarian disease, bladder infection and diseases of the womb (endometriosis). Pain need not always be severe. We appreciate pain in different intensities based on our mood, our experience of the disease we have and how distracted we are. Some women I have met describe their cystitis as a mild abdominal 'headache'. This concept of the 'headache in the pelvis' can seem to trivialize bladder symptoms but low grade pain, after a while, becomes an annoyance and eventually chronic pain becomes depressing. It's no surprise that clinical depression is a feature of recurrent and persisting cystitis.

Blood can appear in acute and chronic bladder infections. Passing blood is a shocking experience and it's no surprise that this is often the trigger for patients to visit the doctor. The urine can range from a normal colour, through rose and even look like pure blood. A surprisingly small amount of blood can look very dramatic mixed with wee. Occasionally clots of blood collect in the bladder and appear as small dark matter in the toilet pan. More often the urine itself if cloudy, 'strong' and smelly.

Cloudiness is often the result of lots of cellular debris being shed into the urine as a result of the infection.

Strong urine is a vague term with different meanings but mostly refers to urine that appears darker in colour, perhaps the result of blood or dehydration. Finally the smell can range from 'musty' to 'fishy' and is characteristic of the growth of the commonest bacteria infect the bladder – e coli.

In fact not any of these 'classical' symptoms are required to establish to diagnosis of cystitis. I would say that 1 in 3 patients patient's with 'atypical' features. Atypical features are more common with recurrent and persisting infection. The key thing to understand with these illnesses is that they are truly 'chronic' disease – illness that goes on and on and on. Because the illness recurs or persists there is little opportunity for the body to return to normal. Valuable infection fighting mechanisms become exhausted and there is a constant drain on energy trying to fight and fend off cystitis. The result is a body that is immuno-depressed, that is prone to other diseases such as the common seasonal viral infections. And when energy levels are low so too is mood.

It is typical for patients with chronic bladder infection and recurrent cystitis to suffer exhaustion and to be emotionally labile. By that I mean tearful! Young women with these symptoms are labeled depressed, older women are labeled as hormonal and men are simply ignored. The truth is that these people are showing the signs we associate with any chronic disease –they are simply tired and can't cope with everyday things. I try to avoid behavioural treatments and antidepressants unless we are dealing with IC. Treating the cystitis gives quicker results.

We know that the bladder has to share its space. Infection in the bladder will always have spill over symptoms. Sometimes the bowels get affected resulting in irritable bowel symptoms, loose stools and even constipation. The ovaries and womb are touching the bladder – recurrent infections can upset the menstrual cycle, stop periods altogether, worsen period pains and even be a cause of infertility. The vagina is separated from the bladder by the thickness of a piece of paper. Its little wonder then that the vagina can feel tender and sex can be painful. I've seen hundreds of women with dyspareunia – painful sexual intercourse – for whom the simple solution was correct treatment of their cystitis!

Men don't have a womb but they do have a prostate. Chronic bladder infection often spills over to the prostate gland – a sponge at the base of the bladder that soaks up bugs. Once the prostate is concomitantly infected then symptoms become more severe and much longer lasting. I'll return to 'chronic prostatitis' in a later chapter.

Finally it's worth remembering that with infection and inflammation there is swelling. The bladder wall becomes swollen with fluid, it appears as blisters to the naked eye. If that swelling is in the wrong place – at the bladder base-then it can actually close over the exit of the bladder. The inability to pass urine is commoner in men that women. In my hospital every week we will admit 5 – 10 men in 'urinary retention' – unable to pee. In a month we'll admit maybe 2 – 3 women in retention secondary to infection. Imagine the pain and distress. You have an inflamed bladder. That bladder is screaming at you. That bladder is saying 'I need a pee and I need it now'. But, you can't urinate, no matter how hard you try. This situation is one of the most distressing symptoms of cystitis.

In essence there is an endless list of possible symptoms from cystitis. I've seen most of them – fitting, headaches, unconsciousness, itchy feet, bad breath, vomiting, nightmares, skin rashes, fevers. Taken in conjunction with the classical symptoms diagnosis is usually easy but when these symptoms present alone it can take months and years to appreciate that the cause is the bladder. I try to educate doctors to be alert to recurrent and persisting cystitis as a chameleon disease – it presents itself in many guises.

4 THE LONG GAME

Acute cystitis is one thing but the long game is another. When symptoms are persistent and recurrent changes occur in the bladder which both alter the symptoms and lessen the chances of cure. Lets examine some basic facts about bacteria and their wiley ways.

The bacteria's aim is to survive and breed in the hostile environment of the bladder. We know that the mainstay of defence from infection is the bladders non-stick surface and the flushing action of peeing. The first thing that bacteria need to do to is to find a safe place to cling on. The perfect region of the bladder for survival is the bladder base. Recall that the embryology of this region is different – its not the shiny smooth stuff of the bladder dome, its rougher and pot holed. Great! This area of the bladder forms a roughly triangular zone radiating like a fan from just inside the water pipe. It happens to be the part of the bladder that is fixed to the vaginal wall in women or the rectal wall in men. It's the bladders anchor in the pelvis.

Given that this bit of the bladder is just inside the entrance it's often the first part of the bladder that the bacteria reach. Remember that these bugs are constantly in and out of the bladder, regardless of hygiene. So there is a nice warm triangular patch of bladder wall to settle on but the bugs need to do more than settle, they need to fix themselves in position. To do they unfurl long tentacles, like an octopus, and use they to stick to the bladder wall cells. If you happen to lack a chemical that distracts the bugs tentacles then you will have a problem – that's about 1 in 10 of us. The arms lock in to position and form a bond with the bladder wall – it's the start of a long game.

At this stage you need to get rid of the bugs and your body mounts a great effort – you need to pee more (more flushing), you raise up some antibacterial cell defences (white blood cells) and you shed some skin cells (hopefully the ones that are sticking to bugs). Most of the time these processes will solve the problem, defeat the invasion and cut short their campaign. Perhaps at this stage you'll get some antibiotics, these will kill the bugs outright – if the drugs are the correct ones, taken for the correct length of time!

So the bugs now get clever – they need more protection and they have a plan. As the bacteria proliferate they start to secrete some slime. It's useful slime, thick and sticky. The slime covers the bacterial layer and provide a protective shield. The slime layer is effective protection from the flushing action of urination, it secures the bacteria from any toxic constituents of urine and it gives a constant and perfect environment for bacterial growth. Now the long game sets in.

Effectively we see a tri-layer or bacterial sandwich forming at the bladder base – the base is the bladder cell wall, the filling is bacteria and the other slice of bread is slime. We call this a BIOFILM and it's the key to understanding and treating recurrent cystitis.

Once we understand the concept of the biofilm then we suddenly start to appreciate the full extent of the problem and several curiosities of cystitis are explained.

1. <u>Every time I go see my doctor with symptoms I get a urine test and they can't find any bacteria.</u> This happens all the time and unfortunately means that many people end up misdiagnosed. The biofilm can easily explain this one. The bacteria in the bladder base are hidden under a slime blanket. It doesn't stop them creating symptoms, irritating the bladder base, using up your energy, making you feel low. It goes without saying that some of the bacteria float free – the jam gets squeezed out – but the vast majority of the bacterial colony are protected. Urinalysis in a laboratory relies on some ancient old rules for diagnosing infection. The lab test cultures the urine (puts a sample on a plate of jelly and allows bacteria to grow). Only if a certain and quite high number of bacteria grow does the test result in a positive. Lower bacteria counts are excluded and patients with slime entrapped bacteria will have much lower counts than someone whose bacteria is floating freely in the bladder. Laboratory tests for cystitis severely underestimate the problem of chronic, lower grade bacterial infection. They fail to make the diagnosis and they disadvantage patients.

In my mind, if the test is performed in a sterile environment (easier said than done) then ANY bacteria growth in the urine is abnormal. Lower levels of bacterial growth should be reported. Instead patients are told – you don't have infection and you don't need treatment.

2. <u>Every time I have sexual intercourse I get an infection</u>. Well you will do if you have a biofilm. Remember that the biofilm is smeared across the bladder base, the same bladder base that's fixed to the front wall of the vagina. Penetrative sexual activity, even inserting tampons, disturbs the biofilm. Bacteria – the jam in the sandwich – are squished out and the free bacteria proliferate and create an acute exacerbation of the infection. Similar phenomenon occur in men who have anal intercourse and sometime in patients who have constipation – the passage of bulky and lumpy feaces through the rectum disturbs the bugs. Acute flares ups of infection ensue.

3. <u>The pain I get is around the end of my urethra or at the tip of my penis</u>. Yes it will be. The biofilm sits on the triangular base of the bladder which is just inside the internal opening on the organ. This area is in continuity with the urethra. Pain due to inflammation in the zone of the bladder is referred forward to the end of the water pipe. This is where the majority of cystitis sufferers experience pain and discomfort – sometimes it drives them to distraction. Previously doctors had thought that the problem was inside the urethra itself (we used to call it 'urethral syndrome') and we'd be obsessed taking swabs of the tubes!

4. <u>I feel fatigued and run down</u>. These are the side effects of chronic disease. It would be perfectly understandable if you had a chronic tooth abscess – sitting in your gum, gnawing away, using your infection fighting

resources. Or a long standing lung infection – we'd feel sympathetic, we'd understand why you were run down. But it seems so different with persisting bladder infections. Patients put on a brave face – there are few, if any, outward signs to attract attention. But the bacterial sandwich is there – this is a long term chronic infection, burning away and ready to flare up at any moment. This is the basis of both recurrent cystitis and persisting cystitis.

In recurrent cystitis the bacteria lay dormant in the bladder base, protected by slime and breeding slowly – probably the rate of reproduction of the bugs matches the rate of bug death. In this situation the main symptom is pain – of the urethral variety and a tendency for infection to recur with minimal provocation – sex, dehydration, constipation. With persisting infection the bugs are growing and the colony expanding – releasing free bacteria into the bladder and resulting in widespread inflammation. Here the symptoms hark back to pelvic pain and increased frequency and urgency.

5. If I have a flare up the doctor gives me antibiotics that don't work. The antibiotics that work in urinary infection are secreted into the urine and attack bacteria. This is a great mechanism of action for a drug that has to kill off free floating bacteria in the bladder. But hold on a moment – in chronic cystitis the bugs are hidden beneath their a blanket of slime. The antibiotics penetrate this layer very poorly and hence cannot eradicate the problem. The typical clinical course is all too familiar – you get worsening bladder symptoms and call into the doctors surgery – you are give 3 to 5 days of high dose antibiotics – they work to reduce the pain and frequency – by day 6 or 7 the symptoms recur – you call back to the doctor – this time its 7 days of a different antibiotic – the symptoms dampen down again – a week later and the pain and frequency return – the doctor is puzzled and does a urine

test – that comes back clear of bacteria – frustration spirals out of control!

6. <u>A urologist has looked in my bladder and said I have 'trigonitis' or squamous metaplasia'</u>. A camera test of the bladder in recurrent cystitis is very revealing. The triangular zone which attracts the bugs and the slime is called the trigone. Inspection of the bladder reveals an abnormal appearance to this region in recurrent cystitis – it looks white and swollen. At times the appearance is rather akin to a snow drift lying over the bladder base. Its difficult to budge this stuff – it appears to be stuck to the bladder wall. This is the biofilm and the bladder reaction to it. Imagine a chronic itch – something that you scratch day after day. Eventually the skin you are scratching will change – it will thicken and take on a callous. The same is true on your feet – constant rubbing of your skin against ill fitting shoes cause a thick build of skin cells. This same phenomenon occurs in the trigone – the constant irritation this time is from the inflammation of the persisting biofilm but the end result is the same – build up of excess cells. These are the appearances of trigonitis and the pathological description is squamous metaplasia.

7. <u>I've heard that untreated I can get bladder cancer from recurrent cystitis.</u> Yes you can. It is one of the saddest aspects of my work that year on year I will see 1 or 2 patients who have had years of inadequately treated infections. The biofilm has set in. The symptoms have made them depressed and their immune system is exhausted. The cellular layer has been irritated and in so doing has stimulated a rogue gene in a rogue cell. The consequence is a form of bladder cancer (squamous cell cancer of the bladder). The same processes underlie lung cancer where the chronic irritant this time is not infection but tobacco smoke. Squamous cell cancers are difficult to treat, they don't respond well to chemotherapy or

radiotherapy. The prognosis of this type of bladder cancer is poorer than other types. These experiences remind me of the importance of treating recurrent and persisting bladder infections aggressively. They also underpin the importance of thorough investigations when symptoms have been lingering for more than a few years. As a general rule I would recommend a camera test of the bladder is an individual has suffered with chronic cystitis symptoms for more than 2 years.

I sincerely hope that you never get to play the long game of cystitis. If you do it's easy to feel as if you are the weaker player. In the next chapters we will explore ways to win that game, either alone or with medical help.

5 TREATMENT AT HOME

A – The Washout Phase. At the first appreciation of symptoms encourage the bladder to do what it does best – expel urine. Increase your fluid intake dramatically and quickly. Consider doubling your average daily fluid intake and in all cases aim for 3-4 litres of fluids. This has 2 important consequences – firstly it will encourage the bladder to empty repeatedly and secondly the fluid dilutes the toxic effects of the infection.

The kidneys filter blood and regulate urine production. They have a remarkable ability to change the rate of pee production depending on the state of 'fullness' of the blood vessels. Rapid drinking will result in large shifts of fluid into the blood stream and this gears up urine production within minutes. The bladder fills rapidly and the signals to urinate come frequently. It may not seem to make much sense to drink lots and so increase one of the classic symptoms of cystitis – frequency. But remember that frequency is on your side – trying to expel the bad guys. Think of the bladder as a dishwasher and the bugs as the slimy food on the plates. The more times the dishwasher spins through the rinse cycle, the cleaner those plates become. Sure, this is going to be a nightmare if you try to carry on life as normal. You are aiming to be passing good volumes of urine every hour or so and planning long trips, concentrating in meetings, and the like will be impracticable. Just accept that the sooner you get the washout phase out of the way the better. It should last about 12 hours.

What to drink? Water is best. Avoid fizzy drinks and carbonated products in general. Stay away from fruit juices (expect lemon juice – see below). Avoid diary drinks like milk and yoghurts. For every cup of coffee or tea drink 2 glasses of water. If you have to drink alcohol drink beer and larger but avoid wine and spirits.

You can improve the rate of urine production still further by taking some natural diuretics (compounds that stimulate urine production). Take these things only in conjunction with plenty of water. There are many products reputedly having diuretic effects. They are often sold to promote apparent rapid weight loss (because you pee a bit extra). The trouble is these compounds have idiosyncratic effects – in other words they work well for some people but not for others. The most reliable cocktails I have seen are lemon water and parsley tea.

To make lemon water simply squeeze out 6 lemons and add to 500 millilitres of water. If drinking that seems like too much of a task then add some sugar but don't make it too sweet. The lemon has a natural diuretic effect and it make reduce crystal formation in urine which in turn speeds up the clearance of the bacteria cells. Parsley tea has to be brewed from a large head of fresh parsley with the addition of a cup of hot water. Let the tea rest for 10 minutes before drinking, It is an acquired taste!

B. The Anti-Inflammatory Phase. You will remember that cystitis causes inflammation and it's the inflammation that causes pain. The most effective anti-inflammatory agents are paracetomol (acetaminophen) and ibuprofen. Take one of these drugs, provided you can safely, at the maximum dose appropriate to your circumstances. And then continue to take them at the recommended dose interval for 24 hours. This is important. You might to start to feel better quickly in the washout phase but the inflammatory effects of the cystitis will last persist longer than the bugs. The drugs will not only deal with pain but will reduce the swelling in the bladder lining – this aids the flush out of the bacteria and also reduces the chances of recurrent infection.

There are a number of alternative anti-inflammatory compounds which may be taken instead of or in compliment to drugs. Here there is more evidence for the effectiveness of these compounds than for the diuretic supplements. I recommend Vitamin E in high dose for 48 hours (take one standard capsule 3 times a day). You can also take omega-3 fish oil capsules at similar dose and again for 48 hours. Whilst there is not much concrete evidence for the long term effects of these supplements there is an overwhelming anti-inflammatory effect in short term use. Vitamin E is excreted into the urine (in other words it is eliminated from the body in pee) and the urine concentrates large amounts of very active byproducts of Vitamin E. Vitamin E becomes a stable diet supplement for chronic cystitis sufferers too.

C. Rest and Recuperation Phase. It seems that most of

us battle on with life when we start to get cystitis symptoms. In the first 24 hours of the illness the body rapidly diverts its attentions to fighting the infection. The result is that a sense of tiredness and exhaustion rapidly takes over. Succumb to the tiredness and rest. That doesn't always mean going to bed but it does mean avoiding physical activity as far as possible. It's also preferable to avoid too much mental strain. If you can postpone engagements, meetings and stressful social encounters then do so immediately. 24 hours of rest and isolation will encourage a speedier recovery and ultimately you'll be giving 100% again within 1 to 2 days. If you resist the temptation to rest then recovery is overall slower and you'll loose physical and mental productivity over a far longer period. Anyway, you'll be peeing so much that you'll not want to stray too far from a toilet!

D. Things to Avoid. I guess because I seen and heard most things with regards to cystitis I've collected a long list of do's and don't. The don't do list is particularly important.

Don't ignore your symptoms. Most people can self diagnose acute cystitis. It's always inconvenient. It's never a good news day! But avoiding the truth will simply end you in more trouble. Pick up the early symptoms and start the 3 phase treatment as soon as possible.

Don't expect too much too soon. You are ill and although there is little to show, urinary infections are serious. You'll need that rest and you need some space to recover. Be selfish, mark out your boundaries and protect yourself.

Don't have any spicy foods, strong alcohol or sex. These things always make the symptoms worse in the first 48 hours and never speed up the recovery.

Don't try to scrub yourself clean. This infection has nothing to do with hygiene. Addition of products to the bath water, over zealous cleaning of the vagina or penis and underwear paranoia will not help you and may actually damage your skin.

Don't get worried about your smell. More women are worried about smelling of urine than you would possibly believe. It is normal for your urine to smell stronger at the start of cystitis but its not possible for that smell to permeate your clothes. Flush the toilet as soon as possible after urinating and the smell will be gone in seconds. It lingers in your own nose than in the air and hence you'll be convinced that you smell – you don't!

Don't hold on. I've heard horror stories of patients being told to hold on when they get the desire to pee in cystitis. I think that there is a belief that holding on might reduce frequency and prevent bad bladder habits in the future. It's just nonsense. When you need to go – go pee. You need your bladder to be empty as much as possible and holding onto infected urine is dangerous.

Don't self medicate with drugs that normally require a prescription. I can search for and obtain just about anything online. But buying drugs is a minefield and you are not doing yourself any favours trying to be your own physician.

Finally and most importantly, don't ignore your symptoms if they persist for longer than 24 hours despite the above treatments. Rapid access to antibiotics therapy is the next stage. Get to see a doctor, don't underplay your symptoms. You are an urgent case!

6 TREATMENT FROM YOUR DOCTORS

I am constantly hearing that the medical fraternity is not sympathetic to the needs of patients with cystitis. Don't be too hard on your doctors!

Cystitis, or UTI (urinary tract infection) as your doctors will call it, is an everyday symptom and diagnosis for a family doctor. And UTI is a protocol driven illness. What does that mean? It means that most countries will have nationally agreed guidelines on the treatment of cystitis. The great thing about guidelines is that it takes away some of the idiosyncratic errors in the treatment of UTI – doctors make less mistakes. The problem with guidelines is that they 'de-personalize' the illness – the human being with the problem (you) becomes a list of symptoms and investigations with a predetermined treatment.

All medical time is expensive – doctors have to speed up and slow down depending on the problem they are faced with. In actual fact most doctors are delighted when you tell them you have urinary frequency and pain – it's an easy win for them! They can speed up the consult and reach the treatment in double quick time – in so doing they've got longer with the next guy who has odd aches and pains and doesn't fit into a neat diagnostic category. And this approach is perfect for acute cystitis – there simply is little else to say or discover. If the doctor is prepared to make the diagnosis based on a urinary dipstick test then you should be leaving the encounter with a prescription for antibiotics.

Antibiotic prescribing is currently in the news practically every week. The key issue is that it's difficult for drug companies to make money from designing, testing and selling new antibiotics. We are increasingly reliant on a rather tired looking stock of drugs that were invented half a decade ago. And the bugs we meet in the world are not stupid cells. We've seen how cunning they are at invading the bladder, well they get a whole lot smarter in the face of drugs designed to kill them! Antibiotic resistance is just a fact of life – it's Darwin's Natural Selection in action – singling out slight variation in the bug structure that makes it survive longer when exposed to an antibiotic. And just like Darwin has proposed for the transition from ape to man, so the transition from one bug to another happens slowly but surely over years. As a consequence we don't have just one type of e. coli bacteria which inhabits the bladder but 100's of strains that could potentially cause infection. It's actually amazing that we still have antibiotics that work!

Urinary infection is one area where antibiotics are essential. There are no corners to cut and the long term health consequences of rationing antibiotic treatment for cystitis is a false economy. By that I mean that if the doctor wants to ration your exposure to antibiotics to treat an acute infection then they run the risk of tipping you into persisting or recurrent disease. Ultimately the patients with chronic infection use up far greater quantities of antibiotics than those with acute cystitis.

There are a reliable handful of drugs that work in the majority of individuals with UTI. The key questions for your doctor centre on decoding your past history, your other health problems, your allergies and your responses to previous antibiotics before making the decision on a single drug. I would never encourage 'self prescribing' however tempting that may seem and however easy it may appear with the emergence of the 'internet pharmacy'. Self prescribing can't make up for years of medical training and, more importantly, many more years of experience on the job.

The main drugs used are:

Nitrofurantoin - usually prescribed for 5 days
Trimethoprim – usually prescribed for 3 days
Flouroquinolone – usually prescribed for 7 days
Penicillin – usually prescribed for 10 days

All of these drugs are known by different names in different countries and many have registered trade names which can make comparison and recommendations difficult. Wherever you may be your doctor will know the generic names given above and they are usually evident in the small print on the packet.

My personal choice is Nitrofurantoin but some individuals are allergic or taking other medication which can cross react with this particular drug. In these cases I would use Trimethoprim. I reserve the flouroquinolone drugs for special cases.

For each of these drugs about 15% of the bugs will be immune – that means that there's a 15% chance that they simply don't work for you. This figure varies country to country and even city to city! You'll know that they are not working if there is no improvement in your symptoms after taking the drug for 24 hours. Yes – 24 hours. That is all it should be taking to get acute cystitis killed off, especially if you've done all the home help advice in chapter 5. So if you are not better by this stage you need A DIFFERENT ANTIBIOTIC – don't wait any longer and persist on getting a consult with your doctor. Increasingly I practice a 'one or the other' prescription. For this I will prescribe 2 different drugs and instruct the patient to stop the first if they are no better by 24 hours and then switch to the second drug – it that way there is no delay.

The urine dipsticks continue to very helpful during treatment. Remember that the nitrates will disappear with the commencement of an effective antibiotic but the white and red blood cells will persist until the inflammation has all gone.

Sometimes you'll just have a bad luck infection. The first antibiotic fails to work, the second makes no difference and you move onto a third or fourth different class of drug. By this stage both you and the doctor are getting desperate and this level of prescribing should be done after the doctor consults with either a urologist or a microbiologist (bug specialist).

Finally do remember to finish the antibiotic course. This is vital even if you feel better by the next day. The temptation is to store the remaining tablets just in case you get another bout of cystitis at a later date. Patients regularly tell me that they have just taken 2 out of the 3 days so that they can take the rest of the pills on holiday! NO, don't do it! Incomplete courses of antibiotics are a major problem which contributes to resistance of bacteria. Essentially you kill of just enough of the bugs to make you feel better but some of the critters are still lurking in your bladder. These ones will be the bugs with partial resistance to the drug and unless you finish off the tablets you are encouraging their survival.

There is more to your medical encounter that just the antibiotics – your doctor will be help you with symptom control. If you've followed my advice you'll be taking anti inflammatory drugs. Great, these will be reducing the swelling and pain from inside the bladder. But pain is complex and we all react differently in the face of it. Some of us will need higher levels of pain control than can be achieved with drugs bought over the counter. You doctor will be familiar with the pain staircase – a simple escalator of pain control drugs that be used until you are essentially pain free. These drugs work in many different ways – sometimes directly within the bladder and other times on the brain and spinal cord. You should be honest with your doctor about pain and get the best relief you can – the severe pain will only last for a few days and so the medication you take will only be minimal. Don't stop taking the anti-inflammatory drugs even if you are prescribed stronger painkillers – they are essential for healing of the bladder.

Next thing to consider is frequency and urgency. I've already emphasized that frequency is good – it's the bodies way of eliminating bladder infection. The problem is that frequency persists secondarily to inflammation in the recovery phase of cystitis. Frequency can become a real chore – it's the symptom that can easily take over your life. We have effective drugs that reduce the number of times you need to pee and dampen the urgency feeling that accompanies them. These drugs are best used short term after the infection itself has cleared. Dipstick tests are again useful – when the nitrates have gone then these drugs are safe to use and can transform your life.

It is curious that doctors don't use these drugs more

often in cystitis – they are safe and have few side effects (dry mouth is common). We use quality of life questionnaires to study the impact of bladder symptoms on patients lives. These questionnaires always show us that frequency and urgency are the main barriers to a happy life in the 7 to 10 days proceeding an infection. I recommend these drugs to start in most patients at 48 hours after the antibiotics have started or when the nitrates have cleared in patients who are monitoring their own urinary dip tests.

So far we've considered 'uncomplicated' cystitis – that is exactly what you think it means – a urinary infection without complications or irregularities. Every so often – about 5 times a year for the average family doctor in the UK, a 'complicated infection' will enter the medical centre. Infections can be complicated either because the causative bug is unusual – in which case antibiotics might simply not work, or because the patient themselves has unusual features – pregnancy, kidney stones, diabetes etc. I will cover some of these 'special groups' in the penultimate chapter.

There are some features of cystitis that will make your doctor stop and listen. If, for example, your pain is 'out of the ordinary', if you have a high fever with sweats or shivers or if there is pain over one or both kidneys.

At this point you could be entering a different ball park altogether. Infection of the blood stream (sepsis) or the kidneys (pyelonephritis) are medical emergencies. The antibiotics required in these cases are high dose and delivered directly into veins. You will need close monitoring in a hospital environment and you'll feel the sickest you've ever felt in your life. If you have these symptoms don't wait till morning to call the doctor!

There is no typical sufferer of cystitis but so far I've

considered the average course of events. Unfortunately our world is not average and there are increasing numbers of people who simply can't complain in the way you and I might do. I'm thinking of the elderly, those with dementia and those loved ones living in care. If you have a friend or relative who 'just isn't right', then always consider a urinary tract infection as the cause. In these cases people can be off food, less mobile or simply more confused than normal. In Europe 1 in 5 admissions to hospital from nursing home residents is due to cystitis and most of these patients have had a delayed diagnosis making their condition and prognosis worse. Don't be afraid to shout out for friends and relatives who are less able to shout for themselves.

Treating cystitis with a two tier approach means that at the first suggestion of symptoms you follow the 24 hour self help program. After 24 hours, if symptoms persist, you see a doctor. Your doctor will know about the antibiotics that you need - you might prompt them to treat your frequency as well. Trust your doctor and work in partnership with them – you both have your health at heart.

7 TREATING CHRONIC CYSTITIS

Treating acute cystitis either at home or with your doctor should be pretty much straightforward. Now lets delve into chronic cystitis (recurrent and persisting infection) and turn some aspects of conventional medicine on their head!

Remember that cystitis either recurs or persists because of two main factors – the bladder fails to empty properly and the bugs are clever at sticking to their base camp. That gives us two important avenues of treatment.

If you suffer with recurrent urinary infection then the chances are that you are not emptying your bladder efficiently. Bladder training has taught us to hold on – it's simply not acceptable to wet yourself or pee in the corner of the room – society wants you to wait, find a toilet or least a bush. The bladder copes with this because it has learnt to adapt – to relax at the same time as filling up. The result is that we can store large amounts of urine, but because we are storing too much the bladder has lost its elasticity.

Modern toilet training has led to recurrent cystitis and a whole lot of other bladder control problems. If the urge to pass urine is suppressed over and over again then the composition of the bladder wall actually starts to change – some of the muscle changes to collagen. This substance is less supple than the muscle and as a result the bladder stops behaving as a perfect 'fill and empty' organ. This loss of elasticity is like a balloon. When the balloon is new and just out of the packet it's form is crisp and clear. Blow it up a few times or blow it up to maximum capacity just the once and you have a different item – it looks saggy and less crisp. The balloon has lost its elasticity and it doesn't recover. The effect of this is that the bladder fails to empty – it might not be by much (20 to 30 millilitres is typical) – but the consequences are significant.

The small volume of retained urine can soon become stale. We used to imagine that this could never happen – after all, like a reservoir, the bladder is constantly turning it's contents over every time we pee. But no, because of the shape of the bladder it's possible that the same small volume of urine sits there, hour after hour – usually close to the bladder base. It starts to tie up when you remember that the bladder base is the site of preferred growth of the bacterial biofilm.

The next problem with the bladder loosing its elasticity is that it doesn't quite force out the urine with the same gusto as it should. We need a rapid urinary flow rate in order to achieve enough friction force over the bladder wall to wash away the biofilms. The result is that an inefficient bladder cannot mount the same amount of friction over the bladder base when it empties. Sticking to the birthday party analogy – if we try to blow out the candles on our birthday cake, but don't have enough 'puff' then the candles stay alight. So, with the bacteria living in their biofilm word, the lack of force from urination leaves

41

them undisturbed.

Most of my patients with recurrent or chronic cystitis have a bladder that just doesn't quite empty and a crucial part of the treatment plan is to regain a better toilet habit. To start to rehabilitate your bladder you will need to invest in a notebook, a plastic measuring jug and a kitchen timer. Simply record some 'urinary observations', over 3 days. Make a list of the time you went for a pee and the volume of wee that you expelled. Ignore any nighttime wee (after you've gone to bed) and try to pick some 'normal' days – not days when your fluid intake or output will be abnormal. The days do not need to consecutive.

Time Went for Pee	Volume of Pee (ml)	
7.20 am		220
12.45 pm		160
4.20 pm		443
9.50 pm		339
7.00 am	220	
11.30 am		278
3.50 pm		188
7.40 pm	190	
7.15 am		375
12.40 pm	290	
5.20 pm		350
10.50 pm	420	

With these figures you have a wealth of information about your personal bladder function.

Lets start by working out your average bladder capacity (this is sometimes known as your functional bladder capacity) – to do this simply add up the figures and divide by the number of times you have passed urine. So, for example, in the chart above, the average bladder capacity is 3473/12 = 289 ml.

Next work out your average storage time – that is the time between wanting to pass urine. Calculate the time elapsed between each pee and find the average. In our example its 2565 mins/9 = 285 mins.

Now we have data we can try to manipulate your habits. You know roughly the volume of urine your bladder likes to hold and roughly how long it can hold on for. We need to initially see both these figures go down. Basically I want you to pee more often and if you do that you'll be urinating smaller volumes each time you pee. To achieve this simply take off 30 minutes from your average storing time and set a timer for that time after each pee – if you don't like the idea of the kitchen timer then use your mobile phone stopwatch. In our example the patient is going to practice 'timed voiding' at 285 mins – 30 minutes = 255 mins (4 hours 15 mins). I would ask them to do this for 2 weeks and then to shave off a further 30 minutes from the timer. By the end of the first month your average store time has gone down by 1 hour and your are passing urine about once extra each day. It's easy to achieve these results. Because you are emptying more regularly your bladder very quickly readjusts its functional volume and after a month you won't need the timer. The bladder is amazingly 'plastic' – it adapts to it's demands. In that short space of time your bladder wall has started to change and the collagen content is reducing, allowing healthy muscle fibres to grow again – your bladder elasticity is returning to health.

Next we have a volume issue. Passing urine more frequently is great for your bladder's elasticity but smaller volumes of urine passed each time are no good for getting up a good friction force. You now need to address fluid intake.

I've already pointed out that there is vast variation in fluid intake and urinary output. Most of this variation is about habit but some is about poor health. For example, if you have kidneys that don't work well you will have a specific fluid need which is less than someone with normal kidney function. For these reasons lets not start to make strict demands on your fluid intake. Instead let us try to increase our personal urine output by 20%. Taking our example above, our patient needs to aim for peeing 285 +20% = 342 ml each time. That translates to increasing fluid intake by 25% (as about 5 % of the additional fluid will be lost in other ways). It's going to be easy. Everytime you take a drink – drink another quarter of that volume in water. Do this after the first month of bladder training is complete.

Now you are peeing more often and your urine volumes are a little higher. The final trick is to learn to expel your urine briskly. To do this you will need to use your abdominal muscle contraction. A good part of the pressure on the bladder during urination comes from the squeeze from abdominal muscles. You need to make these muscles count. Stop for a moment and think about the way you pass urine. If you are a woman my guess is that you don't have to put much effort into urination – you find a toilet, close the door and the rest just happens. Men actually have to try a bit harder. Firstly they need to aim and secondly they need to squeeze muscles harder to expel urine past their prostate.

It is only in relative recent years that we have taken to

the habit of sitting down to urinate. Standing or squatting is the natural stance. Sitting is a position of relaxation – it's comfortable, you can relax all your postural muscles, read a book even fall to sleep. We don't want that! You need to make the passing of urine an active event. To achieve this you need to squat. Squatting just above the toilet rim will keep your abdominal muscles taught and your thigh muscles contracting. The effect of this additional muscle tone is to raise the pressure inside your tummy and pelvis. This pressure is transferred to the bladder – it's like someone giving you an extra squeeze during your wee and the overall effect is a brisker pee. And it's easy to learn to and remember to squat – simply leave up the toilet seat – it's an effective deterrent to sitting down!

If you can't squat (and lets face arthritis in the hips or knees can make that impossible) or if you are male then you'll need to learn something different. In this situation manual squeezing the abdominal wall is effective. In this case, as you pass urine, put both palms on your lower tummy, just either side of your belly button, and push down hard. It sounds easy but it is effective. Continue the squeeze until you have finished peeing.

Both the squat technique and manual squeezing speed up bladder emptying and make it easier to empty your bladder. The friction forces in the bladder increase and the biofilms get peeled away.

No-one will tell you that you are not urinating correctly but these simple manoeuvres are the first step to effective bladder health in recurrent cystitis – pee more often, pee more volume and pee quicker. The bladder is beginning to clean itself out just as nature intended.

Antibiotics are the medical treatment of choice in acute

cystitis but they are also the bedrock of treatment in recurrent and chronic infection. When the symptoms recur or persist then it's simply no use sticking to conventional antibiotic recommendations (high dose, short duration). Now it's time for a different approach. In chronic disease the antibiotic therapy needs to be given over a long, long period – three months typically. Taking twelve weeks of antibiotics at standard dosage would play havoc with your body, it would reduce your immunity to other disease, give you bowel disturbance and fungal infection. For these reasons a low dose approach is essential. Once again there are lots of different antibiotics that work equally well and you doctor will know which one is best suited to you individually. It's worth asking your doctor this low dose, long duration approach to chronic cystitis simply because it is fantastically effective and less than 50% of doctors realize that it's first line treatment. Instead patients are given course after course of ineffective high dose antibiotics. It is worth taking the low dose therapy as a single tablet at night. Many of these drugs are excreted via the bladder and exposure to the bladder overnight can speed up the effect.

The long course of antibiotic effectively clears the bacterial biofilm – I like to think about it as parasitic fish nibbling away at the bacterial ecosystem. Symptoms are vey much improved about half the way through treatment but it's important to stick to 3 months as there is a high relapse rate for shorter courses. In some very severe cases of chronic cystitis I will suggest a six month course of low dose antibiotics.

Antibiotic therapy at low dose is sometimes referred to a prophylaxis – that is a drug which is aiming to prevent an infection. In some respects it is true but what is more accurately happening is that the drug is preventing the chronic disease from acute flare ups – in such a way your natural infection fighting mechanisms have a real chance to attack the chronic disease. I like to call it 'facilitation therapy' – a drug that is facilitating your body to kill the underlying bacteria. In my mind 'prophylactic antibiotic therapy' has a different meaning. Here I use the term to describe taking a single dose of an antibiotic drug at the time when you know you have exposed yourself to cystitis – this is possible to do if you have identified your own trigger factors (sex, dehydration, long travel, stress etc). In such circumstances we can prescribe the use of drugs at the point of exposure (immediately after sex, for example) and this prevents the infection from taking hold. Single antibiotic dose prescribing is controversial but for a minority of patients it is life transforming.

When antibiotics are not advisable or when they have failed to address the problem then we need to consider more invasive methods of treatment. I am an advocate of the bladder washout. This is a simple procedure performed under an anaesthetic whereby the bacterial biofilm is irrigated with a salty solution contained an antibiotic. The flushing effect will eradicate the sugary coat of the biofilm and the antibiotics will penetrate the bacterial layer to kill them. The procedure is sometimes combined with a 'urethral dilatation'. Here the urethra (water pipe) is stretched a small amount. The effect of this is the speed up the passage of urine on peeing – working on the friction effect we've seen above. In general these procedures can bring a rapid resolution to symptoms that have persisted for many months and years. By performing a bladder washout urologists get the opportunity to look inside your bladder. When the effects of the chronic infection have been to leave the bladder wall very swollen then we know that there will be a high chance of re-infection despite washout. In case like this we can advise on post operative courses of low dose antibiotics or chemotherapy.

When I use the term chemotherapy there is occasionally a pause and look of anxiety as the patient assumes that we are talking cancer. But chemotherapy simply means treatment with chemicals. Doctors have a range of chemicals at their disposal which can prove vital in the treatment of chronic cystitis – the glycosaminoglycan (GAG) derivatives. Think of the non-stick pan. This is the bladder lining we are trying to achieve – one in which the bacterial arms and suckers simply cannot get hold. The GAG chemicals effectively provide a barrier between the bladder wall cells and the bacteria – they prevent the biofilm from forming. If we start off with a clean bladder (achieved by either antibiotic treatments, invasive procedures or a combination) then instilling a GAG product into the bladder will maintain the bladders health. Instillation is via a catheter inserted either by a doctor, a nurse or by yourself. The chemical is then poured into the bladder with a large syringe. To achieve a good coating to the bladder wall I like to see patients turning or rolling side to side for 30 minutes before expelling the chemical in their urine.

The GAG chemicals are safe and do not cause side effects, although passing the catheter tube itself may result in some pain and occasional bleeding. One problem with the GAG products is that they are rapidly shed back into the urine. For this reason we advocate that several instillations are performed over a relatively short period – typically six treatments over six weeks. This means that a substantial layer of GAG can build up. This layer is shed over the next 6 weeks, giving about 3 months in total of barrier protection. At this stage the treatment is 'topped up' with a single instillation and thereafter every 2 to 3 months. This regimen is very successful. Some patients find that they require more frequent instillations and learn to judge for themselves when the barrier is wearing too thin. Occasionally less frequent instillations – as little as once every year – can be effective. I sometimes teach patients to self insert the tube and chemical. This is useful when individuals are away from home for long periods or find travel into the hospital or clinic stressful and inconvenient.

Reconstituting the GAG layer in the bladder actually allows the bladder cells something of a rest from the constant strain of infection and inflammation. In so doing the cells become healthier and the tight junction between the cells reform. In that way the GAG replacement treatment may be just a temporary requirement. After a sufficient treatment duration the instillations ca be withdrawn leaving behind a healthy layer of natural bladder cells. The duration and frequency of these treatments is therefore very variable and you should ask for a bespoke plan.

Urologists have other drug cocktails that they are willing to instill into the bladders of patients with chronic infections. We can try antibiotic solutions and steroid solutions. These have a bug killing and anti-inflammatory effect but require medical supervision to ensure that the maximum dosages are not exceeded.

Don't be put off your own self-help solutions in the face of all this 'medical' help. Remember that the pain is due to inflammation and so taking remedies to reduce inflammation will work wonders – paracetomol and ibuprofen again. Vitamin E is essential somewhere in the mix, as is regular rest and nutritious food.

At some point you will need a bladder inspection. The chronic effect of inflammation in the bladder is to induce changes which can result in the growth of cancerous cells. If you have had symptoms for longer than 1 year then a cystoscopy, in my opinion, is obligatory and annually thereafter if the symptoms are not resolved. I am often asked by other doctors and those who pay for healthcare, what is the standard method of investigation the causes of recurrent cystitis. There is no standard – everyone is different. It could be argued that aimed with a pack of urinary dipsticks then most of the diagnosis is made. In men I suggest that they perform a urinary flow rate to ensure that the bladder is emptying adequately. For women we have traditionally performed an ultrasound of the kidneys but the pick up rate for abnormalities of the kidneys is very low – I don't think its essential. Cystoscopy is the key after 12 months of symptoms and even sooner if the diagnosis is in doubt. Equally I am a great advocate of the bladder scan in women – to measure the volume of urine that they retain after peeing. And that's about it – no complex or expensive tests are useful or required.

8 INTERSTITIAL CYSTITIS

Everything so far has been about infection but now we delve into the world of non-infective cystitis. In my clinics for every 99 patients I see with cystitis caused by bugs I will find 1 case of Interstitial Cystitis (IC). The symptoms overlap considerably but there are often a few clues to the diagnosis -

The pain is usually the main feature

There is very frequent passage of small volumes of urine

There is pain of the whole pelvis rather than just the bladder

Symptoms have been prominent for more than a year

Antibiotic courses have never eased the symptoms

Patients have low mood / depression

The problem with IC is that it is all too easily over-diagnosed - this causes problems because over diagnosis diminishes the true sympathy that IC patients deserve. IC is a devastating condition whereby the bladder literally starts to shed it's lining and forms ulcers. The ulcers start small – as tiny gaps between the tightly packed and watertight bladder cells. The gaps allow urine to contact the delicate and sensitive 'submucosa' (the layer of the bladder just beneath the surface cells). The submucosa contains blood vessels and nerve fibres – urine in contact with the nerve fibres is not a great idea. The small gaps enlarge under the influence of the bodies own defence systems – fissures and ulcers start to appear in the bladder lining.

There are a number of theories as to what is going wrong in IC. The list of associated disorders is long and include many 'multi-system' conditions such as fibromyalgia and lupus. It is probable that the bodies immune system is faulty (an auto-immune condition) but a congenital lack of regular adhesions of the bladder cells to the submucosa is also likely.

If you plug IC into any search engine you will be bombarded by sites claiming to help you make the diagnosis and offering tips and help. It is bizarre that such a rare condition has such a popular following. It is often the case with illness that is shunned by conventional medicine that the internet and self-help groups move into the market. And it's not a bad thing! The patient pressure groups have raised the profile of IC and made doctors think about the diagnosis when faced with a patients with bladder symptoms. But a note of caution – it's not as common as the websites will make you believe. The basis of the diagnosis is symptoms questionnaires – with pain as the central symptom, but bladder and pelvic pain has many potential causes. I make the diagnosis on symptoms AND the findings at cystoscopy.

Look into an IC bladder and it is an unhappy site – the bladder is red and ulcerated (unlike with recurrent bacterial cystitis this inflammation has moved away from the bladder base and is widespread). The bladder in IC has small capacity and as it fills up the pain worsens – even patients under an anaesthetic will demonstrate pain during this investigation (increased heart rate for example). What's more, when the bladder fills up it actually starts to tear and bleeds. This bleeding on filling a key characteristic of IC. Biopsy of the bladder wall can be the final piece of the diagnostic jigsaw. The biopsy will show characteristic Mast Cells under the microscope and intense full thickness inflammation.

Mast cells are usually rare in the bladder wall. In IC the Mast cell population has increased 100 fold. Mast cells are responsible for the release of a chemical called histamine. Histamine is associated with pain and inflammation. It is the same chemical released in allergy and hayfever – the chemical that makes your eyes itch and your nose stream.

If you have a diagnosis of IC the first thing to realize is that this is truly a chronic condition – it's not curable in the true sense of the word. But IC is a condition that is very amenable to treatments that lessen the impact. The first group of therapies fall into the self help category, then we have drug treatments, bladder instillations and finally surgery.

The best way to help yourself is to learn what makes your bladder 'tick'. In other words you need to scrutinize when your symptoms are at worst and what factors may have contributed. The list or 'provocative' stimuli is endless but include, commonly:

Having a full bladder
Having sexual intercourse
Menstruating and the days preceding menstruation

Sitting for long periods
Being tired
Drinking alcohol
Eating spicy food
Travel – especially to unfamiliar destinations

Ultimately you need to make your own personal list by reviewing your symptoms over several months. Patterns start to emerge. Sometimes it doesn't help to avoid the symptoms but at least you have can learn to anticipate them and take action to lessen their effect. For example, if you find that your bladder symptoms flare before and during menstruation then you can commence simple anti-inflammatory drugs 2 days prior to your pre-menstrual phase. If you know that travel to a holiday will worsen your IC then plan around that fact – aim to arrive at a time when you can simply go to bed and rest for 12 hours.

If distinct provocative factors worsen your symptoms then avoid or limit exposure – don't drink alcohol, eat bland food, don't sit for long periods etc. Limiting sex is occasionally required but often leads to sexual and relationship problems, so try to pass urine before and after sex, take an anti-inflammatory and change positions during sex to find which is the most comfortable.

Given the importance of the mast cell in IC I regularly advice taking drugs that prevent the release of histamine – antihistamine medication. These are available as once daily tablets for the treatment of hayfever and can be very effective. Again, work out when your symptom will be bad and take an antihistamine tablet a few hours before exposure to the stimulus.

Drink plenty of bland fluid. Avoid specially recommended juices and concoctions. Water is best. In the same way that I have advised treating recurrent cystitis the more you drink and the more frequently you pee then the better your overall symptoms control will be. Don't get too hung up on the urinary frequency – IC sufferers especially can't afford to stretch their bladders too far.

Don't excuse your bladder and don't be afraid to let those around you know that you have a chronic bladder disease. I have fought hard for some patients whose employers simply could not understand why their employee needed to sit near a toilet and have regular toilet breaks. I have written to airline to explain that their customer has IC and will need to in the seat nearest to loo. I've argued that students with IC do need extra time in exams. It's unfortunate that many times it needs a letter from a doctor to make non-IC sufferers understand the limitations that this disease can place on individuals, but we are not a forgiving society when there is little external evidence of an illness.

Sometimes there is visible relief on the faces of patients when we make a diagnosis of IC – often because they had begun to believe that they were imagining their symptoms. At least with a diagnosis it gives you an opportunity to adjust your mind to the facts – this is a chronic illness, it's not going to get better overnight, there will be lots of visits to the doctor and you do need to discuss this with the people around you. The sooner that your friends, relatives, employers and teachers know that you have this illness then the sooner they will begin to adjust your environment.

When it comes to medicine, apart from the drugstore tablets we have discussed there is a whole lot of treatment available. One factor that often co-exists with IC is infection. The IC bladder is a perfect, rich environment for bacteria to grow. Whilst the underlying IC is not due to infection, the acute exacerbations of symptoms are commonly infection driven. When this seems to be the case then rapid access to antibiotics or long term, low dose antibiotics are essential. One problem you will encounter is that having been labeled with IC many doctors will refuse to believe that infection plays any role in your symptoms. The opposite is in fact true. Sensible antibiotic plans are essential and can be life transforming.

Managing the underlying IC comes down to using the GAG chemical instillations which are so useful in recurrent cystitis. Regular and repeated instillations will be required for many years and you will need to find a doctor or hospital department that is geared up to administering these for you. Build up a relationship with your urologist and enter a bladder treatment program as soon as you can. Most urologists will check your progress by way of symptoms questionnaires and the occasional cystoscopy. For many patients an annual bladder review gives us the opportunity to discuss the prospective years management plan.

We have available more specialist bladder instillation treatments – some contain antihistamines, others steroids. Your urologist may recommend a bespoke cocktail of drugs into the bladder. Go with that and trust them.

For very severe attacks of IC we sometimes use systemic steroid treatment – this is similar to asthmatics who need steroid medication at times of greatest stress on their symptoms. Steroids are used sparingly and for short courses.

When it comes to surgery this can take many forms. In IC the bladder tends to become stiff and less elastic. Eventually the volume of urine that the bladder can hold becomes so small that there is hardly any bladder control left. In these cases it can be worthwhile stretching the bladder. This is done in hospital under a general anaesthetic because if does cause pain. The procedure is straightforward but it can result in lots of bleeding afterwards and the urologist will check to ensure that the bladder wall has not been torn.

One effective technique for controlling IC symptoms is to inject tiny amounts of neurotoxin – botulinum – into the bladder wall. The effect can be dramatic in terms of pain control and improves the ability of the bladder to relax and store urine. The process is simple and needs to be repeated roughly twice every year.

In some cases more dramatic action is required. Removal of the whole bladder is called cystectomy. This surgical procedure is pretty dramatic and requires a prolonged operation and hospital stay. It is not without complications but for some sufferers it offers them a chance to be symptoms free. Increasingly this operation is being performed using keyhole and robotic techniques. Once the bladder is removed then urine has no where to go! The options for urination are then broad a bag (urinary diversion) or the formation of a new bladder (neobladder) using intestine. Each of these techniques have advantages and disadvantages. IC patients do well with both and careful consideration needs to be made with your own doctor. It's unlikely that your urologist will suggest such major surgery as the first line in treating your IC. They are seen as 'end of the line' treatments. Increasingly though, with the use of minimally invasive surgery and with better aftercare following surgery, these operations are adopting a new place in the treatment plan. For some patients it is better to get on with major surgery than to face years of chronic illness and the risk of depression if the standard therapies for IC are just not working. For me personally I find it helpful to ask for a second or even third opinion when patients are failing treatments. If 2 or 3 doctors agree that surgery is the best option then I have more confidence in performing it for my patients. If your doctor doesn't offer a second opinion remember that you are perfectly in your rights to ask for it.

IC is special. It takes some time to reach the diagnosis and unlike the other forms of cystitis it is rarely curable. It needs a long term plan, a mix of self-help and doctor care. My best advise of all is to ensure that people around you understand your condition and that you have a sympathetic urologist.

9 CYSTITIS IN SPECIAL GROUPS

We need to consider a number of special situations which need different advice. Everyone is special but these groups might present with different symptoms or need alternative treatments

MEN – previously we have explored some of the fundamental differences between the male and female urinary systems. The essential difference is the penis and the prostate. The effect of the penis is to add length to the urethra making it harder for bacteria to enter the bladder. The result is that men rarely suffer with recurrent cystitis. The prostate, however, acts against us!

The prostate gland is rather like a sponge – it has crevices and tunnels along which bacteria can survive and breed. In fact, the prostate is the perfect bacterial nursery. Infection in the prostate and the ensuing inflammation is very difficult to clear – 'chronic prostatitis' is a miserable condition characterized by pain and urinary symptoms.

The prostate has a habit of growing with age. The effect of this is noticed by all men at some stage – it becomes harder to pee, urine is passed more frequently and often there is a dribble. The prostate is the cork in an upturned bottle – it literally blocks the flow and impedes the emptying of the bladder. In these circumstances, if infection does occur, then it's much harder to clear. For that reason infection in men often requires stronger antibiotics or a longer course of drugs. Occasionally artificial means are employed to clear the blockage – tubes (catheters) are inserted into the bladder to drain off the infected urine. If infection recurs or if the symptoms become chronic then the prostate enlargement is addressed with drugs therapy or surgery. Some men use Saw Palmetto, an extract of palm plants, to ease prostate enlargement – anecdotally it is also helpful in the relief of cystitis symptoms in general.

Men with cystitis should be asked to perform a urinary flow test – it's a simple investigation where the patients drinks lots and passes urine into a urinal measuring flow. In middle aged and older men it is useful for diagnosing prostate enlargement, in younger men it may reveal the presence of a urethral stricture (isolated narrowing of the water pipe). In either case it may reveal a more serious underlying condition that requires surgical treatment.

CHILDREN – Every illness in a child is fraught with anxiety. Urinary infection in children can be devastating with chronic infection leading to developmental delays and kidney failure. Fortunately most doctors are alert to the dangers of cystitis in children and are liberal in their use of antibiotics. And because most children are fundamentally healthy, they tend to recover quickly.

With children we look for a structural cause to the problem – that is a defect with the plumbing of the kidneys and bladder or urethra. These are birth or developmental defects. Typically we find an obstruction in the urethra in baby boys or immaturity of the ureters (connecting the bladder and kidneys) in girls. These structural problems lead to poor clearance of infection from the bladder and sometimes the blockage is severe enough to encourage infected urine 'backwards' towards the kidneys themselves. The effect of infection in the kidney is to cause part of the healthy kidney to die away – a scar develops which in turn attracts more infection.

Structural problems are thankfully picked up early with modern scans. Treatment is either by surgical correction of the abnormality or by long term antibiotic therapy given until the child has grown sufficiently to counteract the problem themselves.

The majority of bladder infections in children are not caused by structural problems – the commonest causes are constipation and unhealthy bladder training. Children get constipated for many different reasons – diet, too little to drink and bad habits. Children also loath toilets! Who wouldn't when the majority of public toilets are dirty and smelly. Many children also get stressed by having to clean themselves after using the toilet. These factors can result in some kids failing to evacuate their bowels as often as they should – constipation results. The heavy, loaded colon then pushes on the bladder, contributing to obstructed and thus increasing the likelihood of cystitis. Simple attention to adequate fluid intake, encouraging children to defecate every day and providing a clean, secure and reassuring toilet environment will all help to solve the problem.

If you have a child with a bladder infection don't try to encourage them with self help therapy. Take them to see a doctor. Swift medical care will ensure that chronic symptoms are averted and any serious underlying conditions picked up speedily.

PREGNANT WOMEN – Urinary tract infection is more common during pregnancy for various reasons. Firstly there is something physical pushing on the bladder – this can again impair the ability of the bladder to function normally and empty efficiently. Secondly, hormonal changes can make the bladder more susceptible to infection.

The infections themselves are no more severe than when you are not pregnant but the consequences are. One off, simple cystitis is unlikely to cause any complications if it is treated quickly but repeated infections can put stress on the unborn baby. If infections become complicated by kidney infection then the results are often failure of the baby to grow correctly, low birth weight and sometimes termination of pregnancy. For these reasons infection in pregnancy should be treated as an emergency and treated by doctors without delay. Antibiotics are safe in pregnancy and occasionally do need to given daily in order to avoid repeat or chronic cystitis. In general, doctors have a lower threshold than normal to treat infection with prophylactic antibiotics in pregnant women.

ELDERLY AND INFIRM – The highest rates of cystitis come in groups of elderly women and infirm individuals. Cystitis is the commonest infection in nursing homes and often these are often the groups who can access medical care least quickly. Infection in the elderly may present in a different way. Patients may not complain of typical symptoms – they may simple not 'be right', off food, more confused or want to withdraw from social events.

The elderly are also more likely to have catheters – these are tubes inserted into the bladder to bypass the normal mechanisms for urination. Catheters are extremely useful pieces of medical equipment but they are used far too often – sometimes as an excuse for more aggressive medical care. It is shocking that catheters are used to treat incontinence, for example – making the urinary leakage easier for the life of carers but placing the patient at very high risk of cystitis. Catheters become infected within days of being inserted into the bladder, there use should be restricted to short term needs. If a catheter has to stay then fluid intake should be geared up to encourage as much urine flow through the tube as possible. Additional vitamin C in the diet and Beta Carotine could help to reduce biofilm formation of the catheter itself. Regular changes of long term catheters should be planned and where possible catheters should be inserted through the skin rather than through the urethra. Repeated infection in patients with long term catheters should be treated aggressively with regular bladder washouts and long term antibiotics. Best of all would be to change from a long term indwelling catheter to intermittent self or carer catheterization whereby a fresh and disposable tube is inserted into the bladder regularly throughout the day to drain the bladder. This process is far superior to having the catheter left inside although it costs far more in terms of time and care requirements. The elderly and infirm need and deserve more time from all of us!

PEOPLE WITH DEMENTIA – Dementia is the epidemic of our time. It seems that if we live long enough we will all suffer some degree of memory loss or cognitive impairment. Dementia affects our ability to maintain a good bladder habit – we tend to forget to urinate or can't cope with finding a toilet. In some cases we loose control of normal bowel actions and find poo in our underwear. This is all compounded because we simply forget to drink.

If our brain reserves are failing us then we need ever ounce of memory to stay alive and alert. Cystitis drains our resources and always worsens our ability to function mentally. Combine dementia and cystitis and we have a viscous cycle of decline.

Patients with memory loss and dementia need constant reminding to drink. Ensure that there is an ample supply of fluids in their immediate vicinity. Find drinks that spark memory, that provide oral stimulation – citrus, tea, lager. Spend time finding out what drinks individual with dementia truly enjoy – they can have very specific requirements that somehow also serve to spark a memory. I have seen patients who would have nothing to drink all day but when offered peach juice or lemonade will guzzle the lot simply because the smells and flavours reminded them of childhood.

Take care to avoid constipation. There is no excuse for serving people with dementia poor diet, ensure that there is ample fibre and provide small but regular meals throughout the day. If there is fecal soiling or urinary incontinence then the best management is regular, very frequent changes of protective clothing or pads. It is a shocking indictment of our time that men and women with dementia are allowed to sit for hours in soiled diapers – we would view such behaviour with our children as abuse!

Finally, patients with dementia will get cystitis but will fail to tell us. They will demonstrate symptoms with lethargy, confusion, emotion and aggression. I firmly believe that we should not wait for such behavioural changes but should be looking out for infection proactively. Such individual should be subject to routine and frequent urinary tests and institutions should have a planned screening program for residents. It is better to put in the time and effort proactively rather than wait for the decline and the subsequent need for hospital therapy. In such a way patients avoid the stress of illness and the confusion which occurs when they are moved to more intensive care facilities.

10 THE BETTER BLADDER PLAN

The purpose of this final chapter is to summarize the plan I propose for a healthy, calm bladder. For some it will be second nature, for others it may provide you with a challenging time to change your habits.

EVERY TIME YOU PEE – Think about how well you are emptying your bladder. Find a toilet that you like! Maybe it's in a particular shop or down the corridor of the office. Perhaps it's somewhere quiet or maybe a toilet that allows you to eavesdrop on conversation. If you are plagued by dirty toilets then carry with you hygiene wipes that will quickly improve your confidence in the facilities! Lock the door, don't get caught out by children running in or the cleaner barging through. If you are male consider urinating in a cubicle rather than at a urinal.

Take your time, there is no rush. Squat over the toilet if you are able. Squeeze your bladder with your abdominal muscles. Celebrate a satisfying urinary flow. Wait for the after drips to settle. Squeeze out the last little bit and pause for 10 seconds before pulling up your underwear. Don't be shy about taking off your pants. Never try to pass urine with pants around your thighs – you simply won't relax enough. Men should avoid peeing over the top of their underwear – take them down and don't kink your penis when you pee!

PASS URINE MORE OFTEN – We have settled on an average frequency of passing urine that is detrimental to our health. Don't hold on. When you need to pee go and find a toilet. Don't be embarrassed by having to pee – we all need to do it, it's not a comedy act or a sign of weakness. Make sure that you are drinking sufficient volumes to keep your desire to pass urine about every 3 hours or so. Look at your urine critically – if it is dark in colour then it is too concentrated – drink more. Avoid dehydration at all cost, plan your activities and trips to include regular drinking. Carry fluids with you. Remind children, the elderly and those less able to drink all day long.

FIGURE OUT YOURSELF WHAT TRIGGERS CYSTITIS – It is different for everyone. Try to eliminate trigger factors and don't be afraid to experiment. Make small changes but make them last – if alcohol is your trigger don't become teetotal – instead reduce your intake or mix alcohol with plain water. If you enjoy the trigger factor then make allowances – anticipate that your bladder will complain after sex or exercise.

EXPERIMENT WITH HERBAL DIURETICS, SUPPLEMENTS AND NON PRESCRIPTION ANTI INFLAMMATORIES – These products will reduce the impact of chronic cystitis and speed up your recovery from acute attacks of infection.

DON'T GO CRAZY ON HYGIENE – We all need to be clean but don't fall into the trap of believing that excessive cleaning of your penis or vagina will have any impact on cystitis. Don't apply products that claim to sterilize your skin!

AVOID CONSTIPATION – Have a healthy and balanced diet that includes fibre and fresh produce.

QUESTION THE NEED FOR A CATHETER – If you are threatened with a tube into the bladder ask why it is necessary and establish when it will be removed.

TALK TO YOUR DOCTOR AND UROLOGIST – Antibiotics have to used with care but they are not demonic drugs. Some people simply do need antibiotics to clear acute infection and many will require prolonged courses. Ask about alternative therapies, enquire about surgical procedures and bladder chemical treatments. Don't think that you are not entitled to a second opinion.

DON'T IGNORE THE UNUSUAL – If you see blood in your pee then talk to someone who can arrange investigations. If bladder starts to act in a strange way – if you wet yourself or can't hold your urine – seek advice. Illness threatens the normal patterns of life, listen to your body.

CELEBRATE A CALM BLADDER – Most of the time we have a healthy bladder, it quietly and efficiently gets on with a vital bodily function. Stop and celebrate that fact from time to time – it is truly an amazing organ.

ABOUT THE AUTHOR

Tim Whittlestone is a Consultant Urologist in Bristol, UK with 15 years experience in treating cystitis. He is a partner in Bristol Urology Associates and Lead Urological Surgeon at North Bristol NHS Trust. Tim's research interests are in the effect of aging on the human bladder.

Printed in Great Britain
by Amazon